21 Days of Transformation

PHASE I IN YOUR JOURNEY TO W.E.L.L.NESS

I0426324

Felicia Redding

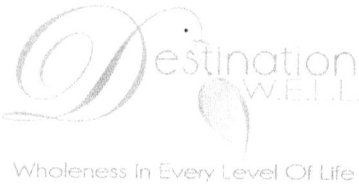

Wholeness In Every Level Of Life

www.destinationwell.org

Destination W.E.L.L.

Lessons Learned from My Journey

21 Day Devotional

Introduction

The journey to W.E.L.L.ness is not only about eating fruit and vegetables, but in realizing who we are and what we need. In 3 John 1:2, God gives us His desire for our health and well-being; *Beloved, I pray that you may prosper in all things and be in health, just as your soul prospers.* I have been reading that scripture for years, but I never really understood what God really desired for my life until now. The reason I only speak about my life is because God has promised us all something different. Isn't that wonderful?!

If I may have a transparent moment with you, I really wrestled with God when He told me to write this devotional. I mean, who am I to tell people how to walk in wholeness? I have so many issues of my own that I struggle with daily. To answer my question, God took me on a journey through the Bible to show me the men and women who had questions similar to mine. Moses, David, Paul and countless others were examples of God's grace. God chose every single one of them, but they all struggled-most in the area in which they were called. Wow! To know that God loves me even when I don't measure up and that He STILL called me to help each and every one of you.

I started this process several times, but it never turned out the way I planned. While listening to a school lecture, my instructor said, 'Tell your story. Most people that are your clients will want to hear about you. That will help them.' So, that's what I aim to do. I plan to tell you my story. It's the lessons that I've learned on my journey. I will not only share with you the lessons I've learned, but personal journal entries that helped me grow during this process.

This 21 day journey is designed not only to challenge you, but to begin the process of creating a new you. A new vision, purpose, and destiny designed to free you. Free you from disease, lack, depression, and unhealthy habits designed to destroy you. I pray that you receive everything that God has purposed for your life.

Are you ready to enter into your Destination W.E.L.L.?

Healthfully yours,

Felicia

Lessons Learned on My Journey

1. **Give yourself a break**-Rome wasn't built in a day, and neither were you! Changes take time. Keep going!
2. **God wants to help you reach your goals!** No matter how insignificant losing weight or fitting into your skinny jeans is, God wants to see you walk victoriously!
3. **There is nothing to fear, but fear itself.** What are you afraid of? You are more courageous than you think. You're moving forward, right?!
4. **You can be healed.** I know you've had to deal with your issue for a while, but enough is enough. Pick up your bed and walk!
5. **It's a matter of the heart.** Once you truly learn to love yourself, you'll want to life a healthier life.
6. **Spread love.** Loving others brings your life into greater focus.
7. **Share your gifts.** We're all good at something, so share it with others. Your talents will bless others and allow you to feel a part of something greater than yourself. Let your light shine!!!
8. **There will be bad days.** Stuff happens. Give yourself 24 hours to grieve, and keep moving forward. Adversity is a normal part of life. How you handle the issues in your life is the most important thing.
9. **Let it go.** It happened and it hurt badly. In order to really be free you have to let it go. Release it, him, her, and them. There is freedom in letting go.
10. **Prayer changes things.** I have heard this said numerous times, but it's true. Prayer will change your life!
11. **Deal with it!** Going through the process of dealing with your issues will not only bless you, but the people around you. They will appreciate a happier you!
12. **Talk about it.** Talking to a professional may be needed. There is no shame in that. Sometimes it's hard to look at ourselves objectively and a second opinion is needed.

13. **Change your mind.** Doing what you've always done hasn't worked so far, so change your mindset!
14. **You're not alone.** There are people in your life that truly love you and want to see you healthy. Don't isolate yourself.
15. **You deserve this.** You were meant to be healthy. You are worthy of living a healthy life. You are deserving of love and everything God has in store for you!
16. **Speak it!** You want it? Speak it in the atmosphere and watch God move!
17. **Stay Positive.** No stinking thinking! As a man thinks in his heart, so is he!
18. **Keep the faith.**
19. **Believe.** It's going to happen, but you have to believe!
20. **Move forward.** No matter what, keep moving forward. It's harder for the enemy to hit a moving target!
21. **Expect the great.** God is going to exceed your expectations! Dream big!

Day One:

God wants to help you reach your goals!

'No matter how insignificant losing weight or fitting into your skinny jeans is, God wants to see you walk victoriously!'

I don't know about you, but sometimes it's hard to believe what God's word says about me. I mean, really! Be honest with yourself. We jump and shout about God's promises in church, but what happens when we get home and are faced with a very present reality? We hear, 'God is going to do it for you in 3 days!' We jump, shout, and run around the church in joy. We declare that we're going to stand on God's word, only to come home to an abusive husband or unruly children. Where's the hope in that?!

Well, let me encourage you. There IS hope for you! Let's look at a scripture that is often quoted among the body of believers: Philippians 4:13 *I can do all things through Christ who strengthens me.* This is one of my favorite scriptures. I quote it when I'm feeling like I can't go another step on the treadmill, when I want a piece of cake, taking a test, or when a co-worker is trying my patience. This is the go to scripture for my life!

Recently my pastor, Bishop Stephen B. Hall, shed some light on this scripture. He said God wants you to do the possible things in your life, and He will do the impossible. I'm sorry if I quoted you wrong Bishop, but that's what I gathered from your Sunday morning message.

I say all of that to say, just take a step towards your goals, and God WILL help you! God wants to cure you from diabetes, heal you from a bad relationship, and help you to love again. The key is you have to do what YOU can do. Not that God needs any help, but doing what's possible increases your faith! When you start walking on that treadmill and you start seeing results, you say to yourself, 'Hey! I can DO this!'

Let's pray about it: *Lord, thank you for this day. Thank you for your many blessings and brand new mercies. God, I need you today. I have things in my life that I feel are bigger than me, but I believe that You are even greater than the obstacles I'm faced with. Father, give me the strength to do all I can to move forward, and increase my faith in the process. My trust is in You, and I believe You will do everything You promised concerning my life. Thank You Lord in advance for doing the impossible in my life!* ***AMEN***.

Healthy Homework: Take some time today and write a list of goals. Separate them into categories: short term-things you can accomplish in the next 1-3 months, and long term-tasks you will accomplish in 3 or more months. Think of ways to reward yourself for accomplishing your goals. Now look in the mirror and say, 'I CAN DO THIS!'

Day Two:

There is nothing to fear, but fear itself.

'What are you afraid of? You are more courageous than you think. You're moving forward, right?!'

Whether its fear of failure or even fear of success, fear can be very real and hinder you from moving forward. My goal today is not to condemn you for being afraid, but it's to encourage you to use this feeling in a positive way. Ok, so you're scared. It happens. However, you don't have to let it rule your life.

What exactly is fear?

Fear can be defined as *a distressing emotion aroused by impending danger, evil, pain, etc., whether the threat is real or imagined; the feeling or condition of being afraid.* The part of this definition that I love the most is that the threat can be real or IMAGINED. Sometimes what we feel and the reality of the situation are two entirely different things. It's up to us to trust God in every situation- even the scary ones. He is there with us to give us the strength to stand tall through every trial.

2 Timothy 1:7 in the **New Living Translation (NLT)** states: [7] *For God has not given us a spirit of fear and timidity, but of power, love, and self-discipline.*

So there is no fear, only faith that God has given you the tools that you need to triumph!

Let's pray about it: *Father, thank You for this day that You've blessed me with. I apologize for letting my fears rule my life. Please give me the strength to walk in the power, love, and self-discipline that You've promised in Your word. Help me to walk in what You've called me to do without fear and to trust You through every task and trial. I love You and I give You all the praise. In Jesus' name I pray, AMEN.*

Tell fear it's FIRED today and walk in the power of God's love!

Healthy Homework: Let today's journal entry focus on any fears that you struggle with and how it has affected your life thus far. After writing, pledge to yourself and to God that you will leave those fears behind and begin to move forward!

Here is a journal entry that helped me express the fear I felt at that time in my life. I pray it helps you deal with and overcome your fears.

March 21, 2007

Alone, hurt, scared, dark. I'm in a black hole I've created for myself. I can see the sunlight coming in from the top and long to come out. I want the Son to warm my face and hands. Especially my feet-they're always cold.

I'm playing games-I'm fooling myself. I'm singing, dancing, and smiling for the crowd. Everyone thinks I'm in the sun, but I'm only in the shadows-I'm on the outskirts of who God really wants me to be. The potential to be great is scary. What if I arrive there and that leaves me too? What if what God has given me isn't enough-I don't measure up? What then? I'm so used to my black hole. It's survival of the fittest here. I tried to peek out and see what life was like in the light and it was too bright, so I just got a sweater and warm socks and jumped back in. It's comfortable here-I've even got ministry here! I'm dancing in the dark, singing and prophesying in the dark. I can only see images of gray though-seeing too much color hurts my eyes. My face is pretty-it's all made up so you can't see my pain. Don't look in my eyes-you'll see my hiding place and you're not invited.

Today I see Your hand reaching for me. It's been there all the time, but other hands covered it up. Deceit, wrong relationships, betrayal, fear, and misunderstandings were in the way. They were all dressed up with faded colors and muted lights. Since I was already in the dark I couldn't see it wasn't You and only those things that were inside of me.

I grew in the dark-stunted growth. I'm still a little girl inside-still holding on to my Daddy's hand and wondering where it went. I looked to Mommy for help, but she's in the hole next to mine. We talk in the dark-never pulling each other to the light.

I've neglected You. I'm such a selfish lover. You are in the dark with me because I was too ashamed to come to the light-I didn't want others to see my defects. You told me I'm beautiful because You made me, but all I see is pain. I hear the taunting from my past, but You're still trying to make me come out in the Son with You. I made excuses before, but now I want to come out. If You can be here in this place with me-this ugly, dark place; then I know You'll be with me in the Son. I'm ready for the journey now…lead me to the light. Warm me with Your glow; make me mature and grow. Let Your love make me blossom into the flower You've designed me to be-full of color, light, and beauty.

Let me reflect Your glory, grace, and speak of Your goodness for many generations to come.

Day Three:

Move forward.

'No matter what, keep moving forward. It's harder for the enemy to hit a moving target!'

Now that you've faced your fears, it's time to move forward. I know, easier said than done, right? Through this process it's been a struggle to move forward for me. The unhealthy habits that I've acquired over the years are familiar to me. Sometimes I think, 'How will I function without the things that I know are harming me? How will I be defined by others if I let this habit go?' Well, I'm learning that moving forward is ok. I believe the same will happen for you! You will discover more about yourself and others around you when you decide to move forward. God's purpose and plan for your life will be revealed to you when you move!

The Bible is the busiest book I've read. It's full of people moving! Noah received instruction from God and **MOVED** on what God said. Abraham was told to leave his countrymen and **GO** to a place that God would show him. Moses was told to **GO** to Egypt to tell Pharaoh to let the Israelites go. Do you think these mighty men of God had questions about what God told them? Of course they did! Even though they had questions, they were obedient to God's word. As they **MOVED**, God's plan for their lives became clearer. It happened for them, and it will happen for you!

If you want to go back to school, **MOVE ON IT!** Do you need to lose weight? Don't just sit there-**MOVE ON IT!** These things that God has purposed in your heart to do are not just things for you to dream and think about. God has chosen you for a specific task to reveal His glory in the earth. He wants to show off His beautiful creation-**YOU!** Now that you have your marching orders, **MOVE** and watch God work on your behalf!

Let's pray about it: *Lord thank You for all that You are in my life. I praise You for a day of brand new mercies and another opportunity to serve You. Father, I want to move forward in the things You've called me to do. Order my steps and lead me to the place You have in store for me. I trust that as I move forward that You will continue to make Your purpose and plan for my life clear. Please remove every hindrance and distraction from my life and place people in my life that are ordained to assist me in my journey toward purpose. I thank You for Your power, my purpose, and Your love. AMEN.*

Healthy Homework: Write in your journal the things that you believe God is calling you to move forward with. Also write any feelings that you have associated with moving forward.

This is a journal entry that I wrote when I felt like giving up. Hopefully you will read this and remember...

April 10, 2008

I remember You, telling me You loved me, making me feel warm inside. Reaching out Your hand and covering me. Brand new mercies overshadowing me, letting me know it's ok to make mistakes, wrapping me in Your grace.

I remember You, speaking of Your plans for me. Opening my eyes, taking me on spiritual journeys that only I can see. Weaving words filled with power, hope, love, and purpose; my lifelong destiny. The earth shakes and trembles with anticipation of the manifestation of Your word taking flight, accomplishing what You sent it to do.

I want to give up, but I remember. I want to be depressed, but I remember. I hear You telling me that I'm beautiful, talented, special and anointed to do an unique task for Your glory. It's hard sometimes, but I know You're here with me-I remember. I hear Your footsteps in front of me. You tread the path, making my way straight. You whisper in my ear, unfolding mysteries and instructions-fuel to keep me going. When my legs are tired, it is Your strength that replaces mine. You love me. You accept me. You bless me. You're healing me. You forgive me.

Day Four:

There will be bad days.

'Stuff happens. Give yourself 24 hours to grieve, and keep moving forward. Adversity is a normal part of life. How you handle the issues in your life is the most important thing.'

Unfortunately, everything in life is not rainbows and unicorns. Although God loves us, it does not prevent tragedies. In fact, the Bible tells us just the opposite will occur. John 16:33 (NKJV) says: *These things I have spoken to you, that in Me you may have peace. In the world you will have tribulation; but be of good cheer, I have overcome the world.*

So now that we know that we will definitely have bad days, how do we cope? I'm glad you asked! We put our trust and hope in the One who has overcome the world! There's not a big secret to getting through a bad day. Just get **THROUGH** it! I used to get through bad days by letting my emotions take control. I would eat food that I knew was bad for me but gave me a sense of comfort. Why do you think they call macaroni & cheese and cake comfort foods? Now just so you won't think I'm perfect, I still indulge in those foods from time to time. The difference is that I don't let my emotions rule my food choices. We will explore that more in the next phase of our journey.

Remember, it's not WHAT you go through; it's HOW you go through. It's ok to mourn. It's ok to give in to your feelings a little. The problem is when you let what you are experiencing rule your emotions and affect your decisions. Whenever you get to the point where you want to do things that are counterproductive, remember the Word. Let God be your strength!

Let's let 2 Corinthians 12:9 (NKJV) be our prayer for today: *And He said to me, "My grace is sufficient for you, for My strength is made perfect in weakness." Therefore most gladly I will rather boast in my infirmities, that the power of Christ may rest upon me.*

God thank You for Your unmatched strength in my life that equips me to conquer every test and trial! AMEN.

Healthy Homework: Writing is therapeutic. Instead of acting on your emotions, take the time to pray and write about how you feel. I believe you will feel better if you give yourself time to think before acting impulsively.

This was a poem that I wrote after an especially bad day...

August 1, 2008

I need to relax, just release my mind. I need to breathe; inhale and exhale Your goodness; leave all my troubles behind.

I'm tired of worrying, tired of stressing, tired of looking over my shoulder. Especially when I know Your presence is a blessing.

It keeps me, You love me, You take on my burdens as Your own; but I'm so stubborn I won't lay them at Your throne.

Today I choose to surrender-You can have all of me. You can have all my problems, concerns, and insecurities.

I choose to trade my ashes for beauty, sorrow for joy, and heaviness for my dancing shoes. I'm looking for Your presence, craving it more and more.

Oh awesome God, thank You for sweet release, but most of all, thank You for YOUR PEACE.

Day Five:

You can be healed!

'I know you've had to deal with your issue for a while, but enough is enough! Pick up your bed and walk!'

The Bible gives us several references for healing. We run to the altar to receive the prayer of a minister and a healing touch; we quote healing scriptures when faced with various infirmities. It's what we have been trained to do. It's what the Word of God says to do. Knowing these things, where is the disconnect? Why are we not walking in our healing? Isaiah 53:5 (NKJV) says, *But He was wounded for our transgressions, He was bruised for our iniquities; The chastisement for our peace was upon Him, and by His stripes we are healed.* Isn't that good news?! Jesus died so that we could LIVE! Our healing was released in His death! So I will ask again, what is the problem? Why are we still sick?

About 12 years ago, my pastor at the time prophesied to me that God was going to heal me from asthma. He prayed for me and laid hands on me. I received the prophecy, high off the emotions of the service. Being a young Christian I was on fire about what God said He was going to do in my life. At the time I was on 10 different medications that I took twice daily to treat the symptoms associated with asthma. I had to get my blood drawn every few days to test the levels of medication in my body, and had to be hooked to a machine daily to test the oxygen saturation levels in my blood. I mean, I was really sick! So to hear from my pastor that God was going to heal me was so awesome! But, life happens and I had a severe asthma episode the next day. It was literally like throwing cold water on a fire. I was done. I said that I would just accept that I would have asthma for the rest of my life and deal with it the best way I could.

Now let's fast forward to present day. I realized a year ago that my healing has been a process. No, it didn't happen instantly, but as the years have gone by I have had to take less and less of the medications prescribed to me. In fact, the only thing I have to use is an emergency inhaler every once in a while. Also, when I realized the connection between food and asthma, it was an eye opener for me. By cutting harmful things out of my diet, I don't have any of the symptoms or issues associated with asthma. The very things I thought were good for me (unhealthy foods) were the things that hindered my healing. That will preach, won't it?! The touch I received on the altar all those years ago started the healing process, but it was up to me to pick up my bed and walk into my healing. Do you have an infirmity? Jesus was wounded so that we could walk in our healing. Pick up your bed and **WALK** today!!!! You can be **HEALED**!!!!

Let's pray about it: *Father I thank You for sending Your Son long ago to die on the cross just for me. I am in awe of Your love and sacrifice on my behalf. Please forgive me for not accepting the healing that You so freely give. Father, show me what I need to change in my life to promote my healing, and help me to walk in my healing from this day forward. I thank You that what I need is in You, and that it is already done according to Your Word. In Jesus' name I pray, AMEN.*

This journal entry was about my dream of being whole.

March 22, 2007

The deepest part of me longs for You. There is a spot that is open-it's incomplete. I tried to close it up on my own. I put spackle and rocks, men, and even food there, but I just became unhealthy. The hole is still there, getting larger by the minute...I'm desperate to be made whole.

What does being whole feel like? What does it look like? What color is it? Does it have a smell? Will I walk differently? What will I say? Will I be taller? Will I finally lose weight? Will my skin clear up? Really God, what will it be like? I'm so excited about the possibilities now. I'm walking towards wholeness. Thank You for leading me and holding my hand because I don't know where wholeness is. Will I sing better? Will I finally be able to leap and dance pointe? The possibilities are endless!

Wholeness is my goal. It's like breaking through the banner at the finish line of a long race. Running a marathon at top speed and never getting tired-no albuterol needed. It's freedom to dance and spin, jump and turn, whirl and skip-it's JOY! It's beauty-fabrics billowing in the wind with colors never seen before. It's well; I don't know because I'm not there yet.

Sometimes I want to turn around though because I don't know if I really want to invest the time it takes. These scabs over my wounds are old. I've had them for a long time. They're rough, but they're old friends. I'm used to looking at them-we have history. They go with me everywhere. That old molestation scar is deep in my skin. Fear is always consistent. I can trust these things. I know I need to walk towards wholeness though, because the walk of the wounded is wearing me out. I'm tired. My legs are heavy from carrying so much weight. I've been walking too long.

I see the beauty under these scars. You've given me a peek and I'm anxious to peel them back and really see what I look like. Who am I really? Do I like cheese and meat? Do I drive fast? Are my feet big? What do You see when You look at me? What's the new me like? Do I like movies? Do I have a new singing voice? Can I play an instrument skillfully? Can I choreograph beautiful dance pieces for a company? Am I an author of a book? Can I own businesses? Yes, I believe I can. You know what? I believe I want to take the scenic route. I want to stroll through and watch You make me. I'll enjoy the day and night alike. I'll enjoy the different colors-pinks, yellows, reds, blues and even grays.

Day Six:

Change your mind.

'Doing what you've always done hasn't worked so far, so change your mindset!'

Now we're getting to the hard part of this journey. You guessed it! Change! We hear this word all the time, and it means something different to each of us. To some it means to go in another direction, or do something we haven't done before. For example, moving to another state, starting a new job, or getting married. Change comes in many shapes, forms, and sizes.

Let's start with defining the word change so we can see it better:

Change is *to cause to be different, or to give a completely different form or appearance to; transform.* So, what does that mean? How can I truly change? I've heard it said many times, the more things change, the more things stay the same. Maybe. I say, let change begin with you. You decided to start this journey because you recognized that change was necessary to move forward. Sometimes those changes can be overwhelming, but let's start with one thing at a time. Do you want a stronger marriage? Lose weight? Start a new career? Let me encourage you! You're moving in the right direction!

I believe God's Word says it best in Romans 12:1-2 (MSG)

1-2 So here's what I want you to do, God helping you: Take your everyday, ordinary life—your sleeping, eating, going-to-work, and walking-around life—and place it before God as an offering. Embracing what God does for you is the best thing you can do for him. Don't become so well-adjusted to your culture that you fit into it without even thinking. Instead, fix your attention on God. You'll be changed from the inside out. Readily recognize what he wants from you, and quickly respond to it. Unlike the culture around you, always dragging you down to its level of immaturity, God brings the best out of you, develops well-formed maturity in you.

Isn't that great?! God is HELPING you through this process!!!

Let's pray about it:

Lord, thank you for this day. Thank you for your many blessings and an opportunity to tell you how great you are! Father, I want to change, but I need your help. Lead me and direct me to those areas in my life that I need to change. I open my heart, mind, and spirit so that I may receive what you have in store for me on this journey. Please give me the strength that I need to move forward and follow your instructions. I thank you in advance for exceeding my expectations .In the matchless name of Jesus I pray, **AMEN**.

Healthy Homework:

Your assignment today is to think about what it is you would like to change in your life, and why. Take some time to meditate and seek the Lord for direction. Write your thoughts in your journal. Remember to think and dream big! Nothing is impossible!!

Day Seven:

Give yourself a break!
'Rome wasn't built in a day and neither were you! Changes take time. Keep going!'

Today's lesson is near and dear to my heart! I have always been my harshest critic. I don't know if it's because I'm the oldest child, or that I'm just a perfectionist. I believe it's a little of both. Since I was a child I have always put pressure on myself to do everything right. As I got older I realized that I was going to have a stroke if I didn't just plain old chill out! Yes, I know you want to meet your wellness goals. Yes, I know that for some of you it's a life and death situation. With that being said, GIVE YOURSELF A BREAK!!!! You didn't become unhealthy overnight, so know that it's going to take some time to reach your goals. Be patient and enjoy the journey!

When I say enjoy the journey, I mean the speed bumps on the road too. You know those speed bumps. That *I can't believe I ate that Snickers* speed bump. The *I told my co-worker off* speed bump. How about the *I missed my workout today* speed bump? What can I say? It happens. Yes, even to me! What you must remember is that we are ALL in the process of becoming what God desires us to be. We are constantly evolving, growing, and changing. It's a part of life. I know you want to be successful, but setbacks are a part of life.

So instead of thinking all is lost, keep going! When you fall off the wellness wagon-I say when because you WILL at least once-get up, dust yourself off and jump right back on!
Romans 8:1 (NKJV) says, *There is therefore now no condemnation to those who are in Christ Jesus, who do not walk according to the flesh, but according to the Spirit.* That's right! What happened is in the past, so let it STAY there!

Let's pray about it: *Father, You are awesome and worthy of all praise. I thank You for being who You are in my life. Thank You for changing my life. Lord, I bind up everything in my life that would try to get me to concentrate on my past. I thank You for forgiving my sins today and for the courage to forgive myself. AMEN.*

Healthy Homework:

Write about any hiccups you have had in your journey thus far. When you're done, take the page(s) and tear it (them) up! What's done is done! Tomorrow is a new day!

Day Eight:

It's a matter of the heart.

'Once you truly learn to love yourself, you'll want to live a healthier life.'

Let's talk about your heart. The heart is an amazing muscle. Although it only weighs 8 to 10 ounces, it's powerful enough to pump blood throughout your entire body. Scientific facts aside, the heart has always been associated with love. You know all about love, right? Most of us have had many experiences with love in our lives. Whether it's the love of your family, your spouse, friends, or fellow church members; love makes the world go round! So what happens when that love is dysfunctional?

God sending Jesus to earth to die for our sins is the best example of love we can ever hope to have. His unselfish sacrifice shows us how to forgive and how to love unconditionally. Easier said than done, right? I hear you asking, 'How do I get past these uncharitable feelings?' I'm glad you asked! The Bible can never steer us wrong. If we ask God to help us, then we can get past the hurt. God wants us to be able to love not only our neighbors freely, but also ourselves. So let's start with a clean slate.

Our prayer today can be found in Psalms 51:7-12:

(NIV) Create in me a pure heart, O God, and renew a steadfast spirit within me.

God can make all things new if we allow Him to. By praying this simple yet profound prayer, we can make one more step in our journey to transformation.

Healthy Homework: As I mentioned earlier, God wants us to be able to love freely. Let's start with ourselves. Write a love letter to yourself. Go all out in your writing. Dig deep down inside and tell yourself how truly wonderful you are. After you write your letter, light some candles, put on

some soft music, stand in the mirror, and read your letter to yourself. This should be easy, because you're awesome right?! Psalm 139:14 (NIV) says, *I praise you because I am fearfully and wonderfully made;*
your works are wonderful, I know that full well. Write in your journal how you felt before and after writing/reading your letter.

This journal entry is one of my favorites! I was loving on myself and my Creator. I pray you enjoy it!

September 13, 2007

Loud. Passionate. Creative. Free. Most folks can't handle me. Full of life, love and possibilities. Full of laughter, hope and mischief. I smile, but my eyes are hidden. I'm thinking of things I can't share with you. I'm letting God take me there. To those places only He can show me. I can see African villages, venues overseas. I am dancing, preaching, and singing. I'm walking in my purpose. I talk to Him when nobody is listening. When we're alone, I sing praises to His name. There is no need to explain my song, because He put it in my spirit. I write with the pen of a ready writer because it's in me. I'm putting all my thoughts on paper forever to be recorded in the Lamb's book of life. He inspires me. He's the reason I live. I dance in this space. Twirling around and around until I lose my breath. No one can stop me here. There is no competition-no battles. This dance is to an audience of one-no one is watching but Him.

He's pleased with me, and I get lost in His presence. He speaks over my soul, making me high off His breath. He makes me smile. My eyes are cast upward, wondering if my faith can reach up there and join Him. Although my leaps aren't technically sound, He gets off His throne and claps His hands. His every wish is my command. He's got me so open all I can see is Him. People walk by and stare and call me strange. They will never understand what we have. Our relationship is unique. I've never experienced another of its kind. I talk to you like I speak to my best friend and You talk back. We have tea together. I am always with You, and You're with me. We're inseparable. You even speak to me when I listen to Stevie, India, Donnie and Will. Even Rachelle and Jill. Most people can't handle that. You're the only one who knows I'm free to be me-a southern belle with a dimpled smile. I'm that tall girl who loves to dance not only to Kirk Franklin, but mellows out to the melodies coming from Coltrane's horn. I believe You join me when I close my eyes and listen to the Elements-the music moving me.

I'm not going to worry about hanging out in this space. One day I'll be able to share this part of me. Until then I will continue to follow the Elements advice....be ever wonderful...stay as you are.

Day Nine:

Spread love.
'Loving others brings your life into greater focus.'

Love, love, and more love! As I stated yesterday, love makes the world go round! As a young girl, I grew up watching love stories like Cinderella and Snow White. These movies taught me that my true love will be a knight in shining armor, coming to rescue me from a life of peril. Although they were entertaining, these fairy tales also gave me an incorrect image of what true love really is. In our present society, we are inundated with images of love every day. We see images of love on television, read about it in books, and encounter our loved ones on a daily basis. Most of our daily interactions with others are based on what we've learned over the years about love. Some of us even use love as a measurement of happiness in our lives. The problem with that is if that love is dysfunctional, it affects your quality of life. Instead of focusing on what we lack in the love department, try spreading love! I mean, isn't loving one another one of the greatest commandments?

The Bible says in Mark 12:30-31, (NIV) *Love the Lord your God with all your heart and with all your soul and with all your mind and with all your strength. The second is this: 'Love your neighbor as yourself.' There is no commandment greater than these."* By following this commandment and focusing your energy on loving someone else is liberating! After all, it's better to GIVE than to receive! Opening your heart up to love others is truly a blessing. Now I'm not asking you to go around and hug random strangers, but I am asking you to smile every once in a while! A genuine smile will not only brighten their day, but yours too! Besides, love is not only about the touchy feely stuff; it's about putting someone else's feelings above your own.

Spread love today by taking an elderly neighbor to the grocery store, or doing yard work. I know you had a long hard day at work, but take some time to play outside with your children. Smile and say hello to that co-worker who never has a kind word to say to you. It will be hard at first, but when you love others, it makes it easier to love yourself. Love also brings healing in your life. After all, life wouldn't be very interesting without love, right?

Let's pray about it: *Father, I thank You for being an awesome God, and loving me when I feel as if I am unworthy of love. I pray today that You will help me to open my heart to others who need my love. Help me to be an example of Your love in the earth; not only today, but every day of my life. Father as I love my neighbor as I love myself, I pray that you would continue to heal me. I thank You that as I love others, You will bring continued clarity of my purpose. I thank You in advance for all that you're doing in my life. In Jesus' name I pray. AMEN.*

Healthy Homework: Now today's assignment should be a no brainer. Yep! You've guessed it! LOVE SOMEBODY! Do something nice for someone else today. Whether it's bringing flowers for your spouse, calling your parents to tell them you love them, or taking your son to the park. I promise you'll be glad that you did!

On this day I just wanted to let God know just how much I loved Him, and to thank Him for loving me!

March 29, 2006

You are salvation, always there, letting me know You care.

Your love is overwhelming, consuming, full, and complete. You fill every void-You're what I was searching for all along. You're music in my ear, the grace in every move I make-You choreograph my existence.

Your breath moves everything around me; even the things I try to hide. You accept and cherish me even when I feel as if I'm worthless. Your love makes me shine. I'm precious to You.

You're my friend. I can talk to You about everything and nothing at the same time. You always listen and tell me secret things of what is to come.

You trust me...I don't know why.

You love me with an unfailing love. You're faithful; You gave me the greatest gift. You died so I could live. While You were dying, You knew I would often hurt, disappoint and make You cry. Thank You for dying for me anyway. You anointed me to speak Your word, but instead of proclaiming Your truth, fear makes me run to pursue my own pleasures.

Through it all, You are still here. You're whispering in my ear, trying to spend time with me, holding my hand, and protecting me from harm.

You are shelter, peace, comfort, joy, love, intimacy, creativity, and life.

You are mine.

Day Ten:

Share your gifts.

'We're all good at something, so share it with others. Your talents will bless others and allow you to feel a part of something greater than yourself. Let your light shine!!!'

The human race is amazing! We're all unique in our own way. No one person is alike. Even identical twins have distinguishing characteristics that set them apart. The same can be said with our gifting and talents. You have a unique set of talents that only YOU can do. Whether it's cooking, sewing, singing, or writing; we all have a place where we fit in society. Don't believe me? Well let's look and see what the Bible says about it in 1 Corinthians 12: 4-6: (NIV) *There are different kinds of gifts, but the same Spirit distributes them. ⁵ There are different kinds of service, but the same Lord. ⁶ There are different kinds of working, but in all of them and in everyone it is the same God at work.*

Having read that passage of scripture, you may be asking, "How do I fit in?" Well, I'm glad you asked! You fit in just by getting to work! If you don't know where to start, ask yourself these questions: What do I like to do? What am I good at? What is the one thing that people come to me for assistance the most? Maybe you're a computer whiz, play an instrument, write beautiful songs and poems, or bake tasty desserts. Whatever it is that you excel in, use it to the Glory of God! I mean, that's why He gave it to you in the first place, right?

When you use your talents to build the Kingdom of God you are abundantly blessed! Now I'm not just talking about at church, but every place that you come in contact with on a regular basis. When you have the right attitude while you're working, your relationship with God will be obvious. That means on your job, at the grocery store, or the gym. Matthew 5:16 (NKJV) says, *Let your light so shine before men, that they may see your good works and glorify your Father in heaven.* Something you may think is insignificant can make a huge impact in not only your own life, but in the lives of others!

Let's pray about it: *Awesome God we praise You today! Thank You for who You are and Your many blessings. Thank You for giving me gifts that I can share with Your people. I ask that You speak to me today and show me the talents that I have that will bless others. I pray that you would remove all fear and allow me to share the gifts You've given me with others. I know that my confidence and strength to share my talent is found in You. Father, help me to be a light that draws many to You. I thank You in advance for using me for Your glory! AMEN.*

Healthy Homework: Write in your journal the talents that you have and ways that you can share it with others.

Day Eleven:

Let it go.

'It happened and it hurt badly. In order to really be free you have to let it go. Release it, him, her, and them. There is freedom in letting go.'

Unfortunately, getting hurt is a normal occurrence in life. Like the song says, tragedies are commonplace. I know some of you have experienced things in your life that have totally altered your outlook on situations and people. Most of us have a lived a full life, and with that comes betrayal, abuse, and unhealthy relationships. Some of it was because of bad decisions, but some incidents were due to others intentionally inflicting pain.

When those unfortunate incidents pop up in our lives, what do we do? Do we become angry or bitter? Do we exact our own type of revenge? I will be honest and tell you that this entry is a difficult one for me. I've experienced pain in my life, some things through no fault of my own. As I have matured, I have come to realize that remaining bitter or angry does not benefit me. It doesn't inflict pain on the one who hurt me either. These negative emotions don't free you; they work together to keep you in bondage! The only way you can truly be free is to let it go with one simple word: FORGIVENESS. I know, easier said than done, right? Well, with God's help you can do it! When you forgive, it not only heals you, but it allows God to forgive you as well! You don't believe me? Don't worry, I have Bible! Luke 11:4 (a) NIV says, *Forgive us our sins, for we also forgive everyone who sins against us.* The same grace that God so unselfishly gives us daily, we are obligated to give to others. We cannot say that we truly have the love of God in our hearts and hold grudges with people who have hurt us! Honestly, the person that you are holding a grudge against probably doesn't even know that they hurt you in the first place!

What I'm really trying to say is, in order for you to truly heal and move forward, you have got to genuinely forgive. It doesn't matter who was wrong or right. People are diagnosed with cancer and other terminal diseases daily because they refuse to let go of emotional baggage. Didn't you know that suppressed negative emotions can make you sick? Negative emotions not only make us sick spiritually, but emotionally, physically, and mentally as well. It may take some time and soul searching, but take the first steps today to forgive. It will get easier as the days go by. I'm a living witness!

Let's pray about it: *Lord I thank You for this new day that You've allowed me to see. Father, today I ask that You would help me to forgive. I release every negative emotion that I have been holding in my Spirit to You today. I forgive every person that has hurt me-intentionally or unintentionally. I pray that You would allow me to extend mercy as You extend mercy to me daily. Please heal me from the pain and allow me to walk in freedom today. I thank You and bless You for Your loving kindness that You have shown towards me. AMEN*

Healthy Homework: Instead of flying off the handle, take a deep breath and extend mercy today!

Day Twelve:

Deal with it!

'Going through the process of dealing with your issues will not only bless you, but the people around you. They will appreciate a happier you!'

Let's pick up our conversation from yesterday. Forgiveness can sometimes be a difficult process, but it must be done. Now that we have the 'forgiveness' ball rolling, let's put it all out on the table. There are issues that have followed us from childhood. Maybe you didn't have the best childhood, or your first love broke your heart. Whatever your issue is, it's time to deal with it. If you don't deal with it, it will follow you into every relationship until you do. Do you wonder why you always end up with the same friends or date the same people? Most of the time it's the same issue, but the name of the person has changed. It's because you have not taken the time to deal with the issues surrounding the initial problem.

For example, your last boyfriend cheated on you. As a result, you suffer from low self-esteem and find it hard to trust others. Instead of dealing with those feelings and receiving healing, you decide to date someone else. This current boyfriend does the same thing on a greater level. Yes, some of the fault lies with him, but ultimately it lies with you. Yes, YOU! After all, the common denominator is YOU! Take some time to get to the heart of the matter. I mean, you don't want to be a bag lady/man, do you? I think Ms. Erykah Badu said it best: *Bag lady you gone hurt your back dragging all them bags like that…*

Refusing to deal with your issues means that you drag them into every human interaction, essentially destroying your chance at a healthy relationship. This not only hurts you, but the persons you are connected to. That is not God's plan for your life. He wants you to be happy, healthy, and whole.

God will continue to bring you face to face with your issues until you decide to trust Him to help you. With God, you are an overcomer! You can overcome any issue! It doesn't matter if you've dealt with it for 5 minutes or 50 years, God can help you. Why?! Because He loves you! Romans 8:37(NKJV) says, *No, in all these things we are more than conquerors through Him who loved us.* I don't know about you, but I'm so glad that God loves me enough to help me deal with my issues.

Let's pray about it: *Father, thank you for loving me enough to allow me to see the dawning of a new day; not only in the natural, but in the Spirit. A new day full of possibilities and Your presence. Lord, you know me from the inside out. You formed me and planned a purpose for my life. In the days and weeks to come, please allow me to see the issues in my life that hinder me from living the life you have ordained for me. I bind fear of the unknown right now in the name of Jesus and embrace Your complete will for my life. I pray that you would touch every relationship in my life. Give me discernment and allow me to see what relationships are unhealthy and give me the strength to walk away from them. God You are so awesome, and I thank you for giving me overcoming power! AMEN.*

Healthy Homework: Take time to evaluate your relationships, and allow God to speak accordingly.

<u>Day Thirteen:</u>

Talk about it.

'Talking to a professional may be needed. There is no shame in that. Sometimes it's hard to look at ourselves objectively and a second opinion is needed.'

In many cultures, especially African American, it is taboo to talk about our issues. We were taught to keep things in the family. If there is a problem, just shake it off and keep moving. Unfortunately, it sometimes is not so easy to shake it off.

Whether it is marital problems, career choices, or disciplining your children, we all have very real issues that can affect our quality of life. It is times like these that a close friend or a professional can step in with a listening ear and sound advice.

Yesterday we started the process of dealing with the issues that plague our lives, so let's take it a step further. I know you've been praying and thinking about how your issues affect your daily lives, but what happens when that's not enough? Well, don't beat yourself up about it. After all, we all need help every now and then. Seeking godly counsel is using wisdom. As much as we would like to think, we don't have super powers like the Avengers, or intuitive powers like a Jedi Knight. Matter of fact, God's word says you're blessed! Psalm 1: 1-3 (NKJV) reads, *Blessed is the man who walks not in the counsel of the ungodly, nor stands in the path of sinners, nor sits in the seat of the scornful; But his delight is in the law of the Lord,   And in His law he meditates day and night. He shall be like a tree planted by the rivers of water that brings forth its fruit in its season, whose leaf also shall not wither; and whatever he does shall prosper.*

I can tell that some of you are still not convinced this is a good idea. I understand. Some of you have been hurt badly by trusting someone with your heart (issues). I want to encourage you that there is safety in wise counsel. Not only will it help you to move forward, but sharing your heart with a professional will allow you to see what you're dealing with in a different light. Proverbs 11:14 says, *Where there is no counsel, the people fall; But in the multitude of counselors there is safety.* If you feel like you have issues that are extremely complicated, find a professional to speak with. They can help you on your road to recovery.

Let's pray about it: *Lord, thank You for this time of transformation. I acknowledge that I can't do everything on my own, and I am nothing without You. Please give me the courage to seek help when I need it. I thank You in advance for total healing and restoration. In the matchless name of Jesus I pray, AMEN.*

Healthy Homework: Seek out wise counsel. It doesn't have to be for your deepest, darkest secrets just yet, but speaking to someone can help to ease your anxiety. We're supposed to bear one another's burdens, remember?

Day Fourteen:

Prayer changes things.

'I have heard this said numerous times, but it's true. Prayer will change your life!'

In this journey called life, we are often faced with obstacles that seem insurmountable. Moving past your mistakes or challenges can be difficult. It seems as if sometimes the day would be better if we turn off the alarm clock and sleep the day away. Unfortunately, you can't run away from life. It keeps moving even if we stand still. While dealing with unemployment, an abusive relationship, destructive past behavior, or a negative report from our physician; how do we remain encouraged? Well, I'm glad you asked! Prayer, prayer, and more prayer!

It's normal to wonder at times how it's all going to work out. Whether you're a new Christian or a seasoned saint who has experienced a myriad of challenges, we all have our seasons of doubt. Instead of becoming trapped in the realm of fear and uncertainty, turn it over to the Lord in prayer! Philippians 4:6 (NKJV) says, *Be anxious for nothing, but in everything by prayer and supplication, with thanksgiving, let your requests be made known to God; and the peace of God, which surpasses all understanding, will guard your hearts and minds through Christ Jesus.* Did you read that?! God says don't worry about it! He has you covered! When you surrender your issues to Him, He will exchange it for His peace.

 It doesn't matter if it's a difficult co-worker, your spouse, dwindling finances, or your children. God wants to hear about every little issue that concerns you! He doesn't only want to rejoice in your triumphs, He wants to dwell with you in your valley experiences also. He wants to be our trusted friend and confidant. 1 Peter 5:7 (NKJV) reads, *Casting all your care upon Him, for He cares for you.* Just take a minute and think about that. We live in a world where most people have an 'every person for themselves' mentality. I think it's wonderful to know that there is someone that is not only all powerful, but is concerned about me! Rest assured that while you are casting your cares upon Him, He is busy working on your behalf.

Your prayer is not only changing your circumstances, but it's changing YOU! Your prayers are bringing understanding, healing, and peace to your situation.

Let's pray about it: *Lord, thank You for another day. Today I exchange my strength for Yours, and cast all my cares upon You. I believe that You're able to handle every situation of my life, and for that I am eternally grateful. Thank You Lord for being a trusted friend, and for the growth that I am already seeing in my life. In Jesus' name I pray, AMEN.*

Healthy Homework: Do you even have to guess what your assignment is today? Pray, pray, PRAY! Write in your journal about how you feel before and after your prayer sessions. Be sure to write anything down that the Lord shares with you during your time together.

This prayer may seem a little unconventional to you, but it's a conversation between me and God. I mean, that's what prayer is supposed to be, right?

October 6, 2007

You are high above the heavens, singing over my soul. I hear the music so clear it's surrounding me. I'm hearing You. My ears are open in anticipation, just listening. I hear the distinct notes of the piano, the harp, and percussion. It's providing a rhythm I can dance to. It's telling of what is to come. It's speaking for You. Inaudible instruction, the plans You have for me. It's opening my eyes, allowing me to see clearly. It's moving me, making me raise my arms and sway to the beat. I feel Your song in every part of me. I'm twirling around, spinning out of control. I feel Your love, Your peace, and I'm staying in Your flow. I want to tell the world of Your goodness-You're always faithful.

You're ministering to me. You're filling me up cause I'm empty. I'm desperate for You and I thank You for making an appearance. You make me feel special. You composed this song just for me to feel Your love. Could I possibly be more in love with you? I didn't think it was possible. I wake up and You're with me. You tuck me in when I go to sleep. I hear Your song for me, even when I dream. You dance with me. You make me feel like I can do anything. You hold me close and because the song is so loud, You whisper in my ear. It's just me and You, alone so no one can hear. How amazing is that? You're taking the time out of Your busy schedule to talk to me. You say there's no other place You'd rather be. The feeling is mutual. I'm caught up in Your love. Your face is captivating me. Even when I thought I messed up, You're still coming to see about me. You reassure me, Your melody redeems me. I'm free, no longer bound. I'm able to run and share my story.

Oh sweet Savior, never go. I'd die if You left. I never would be able to survive without Your touch. Just when I lose my confidence, Your song plays louder, spilling over me. It settles my spirit. It provides stability. It keeps me sane, allowing me to trust. You've never failed me yet. I hear Your song in my heart. I'm going to keep on dancing and see what tomorrow brings...

Day Fifteen:

You're not alone.

'There are people in your life that truly love you and want to see you healthy. Don't isolate yourself.'

There is a saying that no man is an island. You can't truly live without others. While that may be true, sometimes I think it would be a lot easier to become a hermit. You wouldn't have to deal with foolishness, drama, betrayal, heartache, or other things that come along with blending with other personalities and behaviors. On the other hand, life would be very uninteresting and lonely.

I remember when I was younger; it was an instant self-esteem boost to have a lot of friends. It meant I was popular, and people wanted to be in my space. I wish I understood this passage of scripture back then. Proverbs 18:24 (NIV) reads, *One who has unreliable friends soon comes to ruin, but there is a friend who sticks closer than a brother.* I really got it twisted, huh? Being Miss Popularity boosted my self-esteem, but it also brought a lot of heartache and drama. Now don't misunderstand me; I'm not saying to shun all people for the sake of self-preservation. What I'm saying is that having people in your life can make your life rich and colorful if you choose wisely.

I truly believe that it's hard to connect with others sometimes, due to the fact that we are all flawed. We are all dealing with past hurts and current circumstances that make it difficult to interact with others on occasion. When everything in your life is unhealthy, (people, relationships, behavior), then it's easy to become comfortable in dysfunction. If you ever need an example of a healthy friendship in your life, consider your relationship with God. Some of us have never had a healthy relationship in our lives until we came face to face with Jesus and His sacrifice for us.

A healthy relationship should be one that is parallel with God's love for us. You should be comfortable in your own skin and free to share who you are-the good and bad. A friend should encourage you to grow, edifying and admonishing you with the word of the Lord concerning you. That's right! A real friend should also be able to tell you **the truth**!

God designed relationships to support, strengthen, and heal you. You don't believe me? I've got Bible! Ecclesiastes 4:9-10 (NKJV) says, *Two are better than one, Because they have a good reward for their labor. For if they fall, one will lift up his companion. But woe to him who is alone when he falls, For he has no one to help him up.* Remember, you're not a superhero! You need help to stand firm in this journey called life.

Let's pray about it: *Father, thank You for always being there for me and for never leaving me alone. Today, help me to open my heart to people around me that can assist me on my journey. Let their concern and love for me be a healing balm to my hurting heart. I thank You in advance for new healthy relationships, and healing relationships currently in my life that are broken. In Jesus' name I pray, AMEN.*

Healthy Homework: Take a mental inventory of the relationships in your life, and journal about how they can change for the better. Also, journal about what you think a healthy relationship should be.

Here's another journal entry that is near and dear to my heart...

April 15, 2012

Hi Lord, it's me. As always, I need You. Like a flower needs rain, and the grass needs sun, I need You. You are my very best friend. I can talk to You about anything. You're honest with me. You give me the hard truth. You wipe my tears and make me smile. You're so good to me! You wake me up daily and grant me brand new mercies-like a warm hug on a chilly day. You speak to me, telling me secrets; weaving mysteries of times unknown. I'm honored that You decided to share it with me.

I'm on a journey, traveling through time. I'm praying I reach my destination. Just when I think I can unpack my bags and hang my hat, You whisper in my ear to keep moving. I'm always walking forward and never looking back. The past fades away to memories of gray and black. I'm moving with Your cloud and I feel the Son's rays on my back. I see Your promise for me on the horizon, so I pick up my pace. I feel Your wind blowing and pushing me to my blessed place.

I'm looking forward to what You're doing in my life and the places You're taking me. The maturity and growth I see. I've come a long way. Thank You for taking the time to develop and prepare me for what is to come.

Day Sixteen:

Speak it!

'You want it? Speak it in the atmosphere and watch God move!'

Your words are powerful. A compliment can boost someone's self-esteem, and an insult can hurt them for years to come. The tongue is so small in comparison with the rest of your body, but it can cause lifelong damage. Blessings or curses dwell in your mouth. You can build a home with your hands and tear it down in an instant by what you say. Proverbs 18:21 (NKJV) says, *Death and life are in the power of the tongue, And those who love it will eat its fruit.* Imagine that!

What you speak in the atmosphere is so important. Yes, God already has your life mapped out, but your words are active contributors to your destiny. So what does that mean? Well, it's simple. You shape your world by the things you say. This also applies to our prayer lives. Mark 11:24 (NKJV) says, *Therefore I tell you, whatever you ask for in prayer, believe that you have received it, and it will be yours.* When I read this verse I was in awe! Most of us are fine with whatever comes our way. It does not matter if those things are good or bad, we just accept it as our lot in life. One of my favorite worship songs even proclaims this message: *Whatever my lot, thou hast taught me to say, it is well, it is well with my soul!*

Now there's nothing wrong with that, but let's choose to look at things another way. Maybe you haven't received what you want in life because you're too afraid to say it! If you're praying for a spouse, don't just say, 'God send me a mate.' Be specific! Give Him something to work with! Yes, God knows your desires, but speaking your desires out loud ignites your faith! What do you want God to do in your life? Speak it in the atmosphere and watch God move on your behalf!

Let's pray about it: *Father thank You for another day full of promises and brand new mercies. On this day, help me to guard my tongue. I want to speak things that not only bless me, but everyone around me. Give me the courage to speak Your word in the atmosphere concerning my life. Thank You for changing my life in record time! In Jesus' name I pray, AMEN.*

Healthy Homework: I'm sure today's assignment is a no-brainer. Journal about one thing you would like God to do in your life in the very near future. Make a list of why you want this to come to pass and be specific about your desires.

Day Seventeen:

Stay Positive.

'No stinking thinking! As a man thinks in his heart, so is he...or she!'

I know Pat Benatar sings that Love is a Battlefield, but I beg to differ. Your mind is a battlefield. It will reinforce destructive behavior, or motivate you to change it. So let me start today by asking you a question: What is on your mind? We discussed earlier that what we say is important, but what you think is just as vital to your progress.

Some of us can trace our negative thinking back to our families. If you were always told that you were never going to amount to anything, or that you're not smart, it's easy to adopt those types of behaviors. For example, you won't even attempt to go to college because you're not smart, right? It is a struggle to remain positive in a world full of negativity. Instead of taking that into your spirit, begin to rehearse in your mind what God says about you. You're not unattractive; you're fearfully and wonderfully made! You're not poor; you're a lender and not a borrower! Take God's word and counteract the negativity! You know what has helped me to stay on my journey? I am determined to keep a positive attitude. I have discovered that most people criticize what they don't understand. Proverbs 23:7 (NKJV) reads, *For as he thinks in his heart, so is he.* No matter what anyone says to me about taking a different path, I know in my heart who God has created me to be. What God thinks about me motivates me to keep moving forward. Today, take this scripture and let it sink down in your spirit. Think about all the positive changes you're making and how good you feel. You are brave. You are strong. You are changing, and I'm so proud of you!

Let's pray about it: *What an honor and privilege it is to speak with You today! Thank you for always being a light in a world filled with darkness. Today I praise You for the fact that I am fearfully and wonderfully made. Help me to be positive when everything around me is negative. Thank You for allowing Your light to shine through me today so that I may encourage others on this road to wellness. I love you. All glory and honor belongs to You! AMEN.*

Healthy Homework: Think of areas in your life where your thoughts have become negative. What can you do to turn those thoughts around?

Day Eighteen:

Keep the faith!

'I know it's hard to see right now, but its going all according to God's plan!'

Throughout my walk with God I've always heard about faith. I read it about in God's word, hear about it while the Word of God is being preached, and many songs have been inspired by faith. Faith is a small word-only 5 letters, but it packs a lot of power. So, what exactly IS faith?

Faith is defined as *confidence or trust in a person or thing; belief that is not based on proof.* Simply put, faith is just plain old believing without seeing. I believe God exists. I've never seen Him with my eyes, but I choose to believe He lives. I believe He can do anything! That's faith.

If we look at Hebrews 11:1(NKJV), we can go a step further: *Now faith is the substance of things hoped for, the evidence of things not seen.* I know it seems as if your dreams are taking forever to come to pass, but be encouraged! God is still working on your behalf! He is setting the stage to ensure that your blessing is perfect! Continue to trust His timing. I promise He won't let you down. That's the perfect example of faith, right?!

To bring this point home, I will share another personal story with you. I am not the typical bright-eyed and bushy-tailed college graduate. I did not graduate college until I was the ripe old age of 33. I remember when I went to my Navy exit interview and the Command Master Chief asked me, 'What do you intend to do when you get out of the Navy?' I replied, 'I'm going to graduate from college and start my career.' He proceeded to give me very disheartening statistics about veterans who start college but never finish. I didn't start college right away, but I kept the faith that I would get an opportunity to continue my education. God even gave me a vision of me at my college graduation, so I knew it was going to happen. My opportunity to finish came several years later and was much unexpected. My college days were difficult, but I believed that God would pull me through. I experienced God in a way that I didn't know was possible. When my financial aid ran out, He made miracles happen! My college days didn't happen the way I wanted them to, but I'm so glad they happened the way God wanted them to! When I walked across that stage in December 2009, I knew it was God and my faith in Him that allowed me to reach my goal.

What do you believe God for? Keep the faith!

Let's pray about it: *God I believe in You. You are so awesome and I am amazed at all that You are in my life. Father, I stand in faith that You are able to do everything that You have spoken concerning my life. As You work, I'm going to wait with expectation. Thank You Lord! AMEN.*

Healthy Homework: If God did everything today that He promised concerning you, what would you do? Write about your reaction in your journal.

Day Nineteen:

Believe.

'It's going to happen, but you have to believe!'

Life is full of contradictions. There are circumstances in your life that will lead you to believe that nothing positive will ever happen. I know God said that He was going to improve your finances, but how can you believe that when you're always broke? How do you believe when presently everything is the exact opposite? The answer to this question is simple: JUST BELIEVE! Mark 9:23 (NKJV) reads, *Jesus said to him, "If you can believe, all things are possible to him who believes."*

Over the past few days we have discussed having faith and staying positive throughout life's challenges. Today is no different. If you don't really believe that God can help you to stay healthy, find a job, or go back to school, then what's the point?! I mean, that's what people call Christians: BELIEVERS! So instead of focusing on what you don't see happening in your life, focus on what God said is going to happen! If God said it, then it's a done deal! If God said He's going to help you go back to school, then begin making moves in your life to prepare yourself for what God has spoken concerning you! That means start researching schools, complete a FAFSA form, and go get school supplies. If God has promised that He is going to heal your body, then start acting like you're healed!

I'm glad that God blesses us with people we can rely on throughout our lives, but I'm extremely grateful that God is faithful concerning His promises. Philippians 1:6 (NKJV) encourages me when I feel doubt creeping in: *being confident of this very thing, that He who has begun a good work in you will complete it until the day of Jesus Christ.* Trust and believe God with all your might! He's going to make it worth your while!

Let's pray about it: *Lord, thank You for being faithful to me when I am unfaithful to You. Father, help me day by day to trust You more and more. I choose to believe Your word concerning me. I know that You're going to do exactly what You said! I praise You in advance for working all things out for my good! AMEN.*

Healthy Homework: Find scriptures that reinforce your belief in what God has spoken concerning you. If you don't know what God's purpose is for your life, ASK!

You deserve this!

'You were meant to be healthy. You are worthy of living a healthy life. You are deserving of love and everything God has in store for you!'

Sometimes it's hard to believe that you deserve to live a full and healthy life. I mean, do you even KNOW a person that is healthy? Sure, there are people all around us that LOOK healthy; but I'm sure if you took the time to speak with them you would soon discover that you were mistaken. Our society has taught us that being healthy is to look physically attractive, earn a high income while surrounding yourself with material things. This teaching is false and full of smoke and mirrors! Many of us have distorted the image of being healthy in our minds so much that we feel that this goal is simply not attainable. The devil is a LIAR! It is God's desire that we are healthy in every area of our lives.

I'm going to be transparent (again) with you. When I started making positive changes in my life, I felt guilty. Yes! I felt guilty! It seemed like the better I felt, the more people around me experienced challenges in their lives. I would think why am I so happy while everyone else is miserable? What is it about me that makes me so special? My guilty feelings became so bad that I began to hide God's blessings from the people in my life. My reasoning behind this was that I didn't want anyone to feel bad about what God was doing in and through me. If a friend called me to talk about a problem, the last thing I wanted to do was talk about how God was blessing me. I mean, how insensitive is that?

God finally got tired of my foolishness and tapped me on my shoulder. He said, the people that truly love you want you to be happy Felicia. I'm blessing you so that the people around you can see how good I am! I'm using you as a living testimony! Isn't that awesome?! To further reinforce how awesome God is, let's look at James 1:17(NIV): *Every good and perfect gift is from above, coming down from the Father of the heavenly lights, who does not change like shifting shadows.* God truly wants to bless you. Not because you've done everything right, but because that's just who He is! Embrace the fact that God wants to give you your heart's desire. He wants to bless you beyond measure. You deserve to smile. You deserve to laugh. You deserve to be healthy. You deserve to be loved. You deserve all of God's richest blessings!

Let's pray about it: *Father, I don't have anything really eloquent to say. I just really want to take this time to tell you two words: THANK YOU. Thank You for all You are, for all You do, and for all You are doing in my life. Thank You for letting me know today that I'm worthy of all You have designed for my life. AMEN.*

Healthy Homework: Write in your journal about your feelings regarding today's discussion. Also, think about areas in your life where you have short-changed yourself and work on changing that.

Day Twenty-One:

Expect the great!

'God is going to exceed your expectations! Dream big!'

I remember being so excited that I couldn't sleep on Christmas Eve as a child. Mom outdid herself as usual, and our home was decorated beautifully. There were so many presents under our tree that they were stacked on top of each other. My level of expectation was heightened not only because Christmas was the following day, but because I remembered how wonderful the last Christmas was. You see, Christmas and I had history! I also trusted in the fact that my Mom loved me and was consistently providing me with what I wanted and needed. My dreams were filled with visions of Barbie dolls, cute clothes, and joy.

As I matured, I realized that our expectations are sometimes met with disappointment. The harsh reality is that people can often fail to meet our expectations. This reality can make it difficult to dream, or to expect that things in our lives can change. Although people can fail, I'm glad to know that God can NEVER fail! He is consistent, and we can expect that He will fulfill His plan concerning us. When I started my journey, my expectations were simple. I wanted to lose weight and become a happier person. I wanted my smile to not only reach my eyes, but my heart. I didn't think that those goals would be hard to attain. The funny thing about expectations is that sometimes we set the bar too low. Our expectations are often based on the disappointments we have experienced in the past. The sting of rejection and disappointment prevents us from trusting God with our dreams. I used to think, I will be satisfied with whatever I receive. Although I realize that what God brings in my life is by His design, there is another level of faith that God wants us all to reach.

God wants to surpass your expectations. As a matter of fact, He can EXCEED our expectations! Ephesians 3:20 (NKJV) reads, *Now to Him who is able to do exceedingly abundantly above all that we ask or think, according to the power that works in us.* God wants to blow your mind! I only wanted to lose weight so that I could fit into a pair of skinny jeans, but God wanted me to design a curriculum to help millions become healthier! It's amazing how God works! I'm sure we will never understand His ways this side of heaven, but that is what makes the journey exciting! Trust God with your dreams, and watch Him exceed them all!

Let's pray about it: *Father, thank You for allowing me to complete this first level of my journey. Thank you for revealing things about myself that I need to change, and for helping me start the healing process in my life. I trust You to continue to help me as I move forward; not only because I ask, but because You are faithful to complete the work You've started in me. Thank You for increasing and exceeding my expectations! I love You and give You all the praise! In the mighty name of Jesus, AMEN.*

Healthy Homework: Take a deep breath, and look back over what you've accomplished these 3 weeks. I'm so proud of you!!! Write your feelings in your journal and take some time to reward yourself.

Destination W.E.L.L.

Lessons Learned from My Journey

21 Day Devotional

Acknowledgements:

Thank you, thank you, THANK YOU for taking the time to take the first phase of this journey with me! This devotional is near and dear to my heart, because it is the birthing of me! It is the beginning of God's manifestation of the promises He has made concerning me. So, my first heartfelt thank you is to the man Himself! He is Alpha, Omega, and the Master of my destiny. I stand in awe of Him daily and am looking forward to the rest of this journey that He has planned for me.

I know this is so cliché, but I want to thank my Mama for just being her! Deborah J. Dixon, thank you for always having my back and for being God's example of consistency on this earth for me. I love you! God blessed me with two fathers because He knew I needed a little extra in my life. My biological father, Timothy Redding, is a special guy. I want to thank him for giving me a love for the creative arts, my long legs, and for telling me that garlic will cure anything! Ha! To my step-father Johnny Dixon, thank you for allowing God to use you to pour into me when I wanted to give up. Your courage to change your life for the better inspires me daily. I'm truly blessed for having you in my life.

Miyako, Twannekia and Tonya: You ladies are the definition of true friends to me. You support me, tell me the truth, and make me laugh on a daily basis. You guys dig my brand of crazy and I appreciate you for it! Thank you for seeing what God sees in me and encouraging me to follow my dreams.

You are my biggest cheerleader. You love me for who I am and celebrate my accomplishments. You encourage me, minister to me, make me laugh uncontrollably and give the best hugs! Thank you for being a man after

God's own heart and for being my best friend. I love you Care Bear, you ROCK!

I would like to sincerely thank every person that hurt, betrayed, and underestimated me. Your rejection pushed me into my destiny. Thank you for cooperating with God's plan! I forgive each and every one of you and pray God's richest blessings upon your life.

Thank you to Bishop Stephen Hall and the Rhema Christian Fellowship family in Decatur, Ga. Bishop you read my mail every Sunday and I appreciate it! I still think you have hidden cameras in my house to record my conversations sometimes, but I love you anyway! ☺

To each reader of this devotional thank you for indulging me. My closest friends know that I am a very private person, but writing this devotional allowed me to step out of my comfort zone and be transparent. I let you guys all up in my business! Ha! I pray that the first phase of this curriculum blessed you and motivated you to continue on your journey. Stay tuned...the best is yet to come!

Healthfully yours,

Felicia

Sources:

All Bible verses were found in: *BibleGateway.com: A Searchable Online Bible in over 100 Versions and 50 Languages.* N.p., n.d. Web. 12 Dec. 2012. <http://www.biblegateway.com/>.

Definitions were found in: "Dictionary, Encyclopedia and Thesaurus." *The Free Dictionary.* Farlex, n.d. Web. 12 Dec. 2012

www.ingramcontent.com/pod-product-compliance
Lightning Source LLC
Chambersburg PA
CBHW070819290526
45795CB00002B/775